Manuka Honey –
One of Nature's Miracles

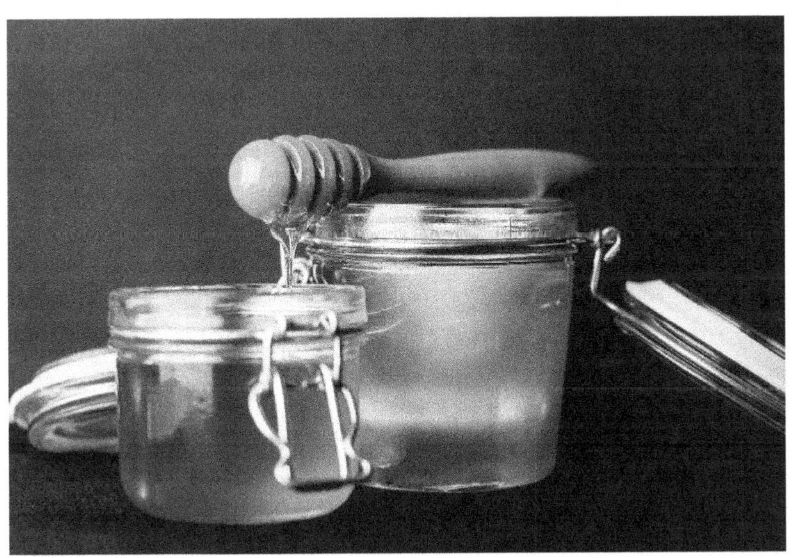

Graham Hodson

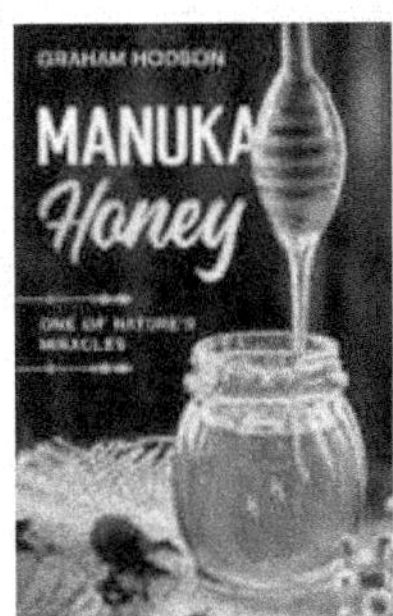

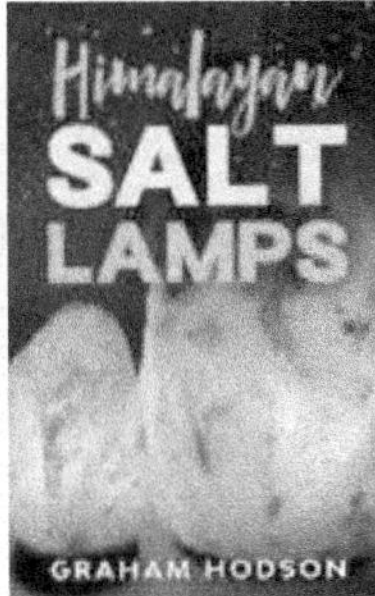

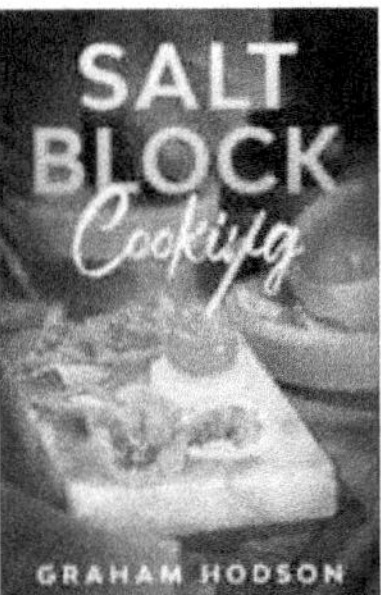

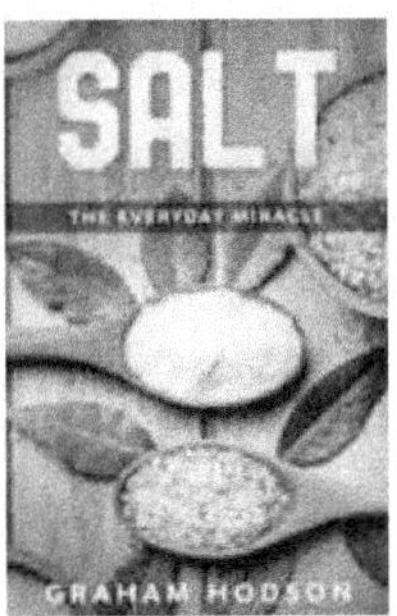

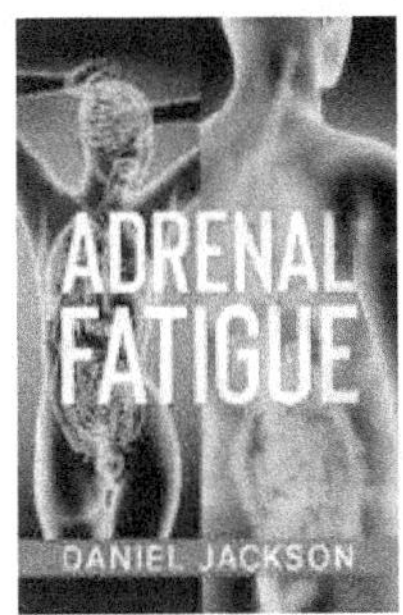

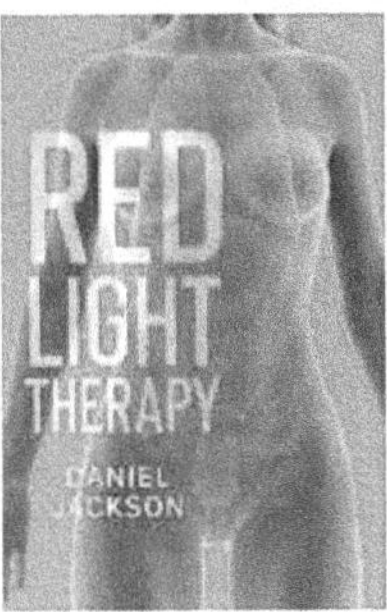

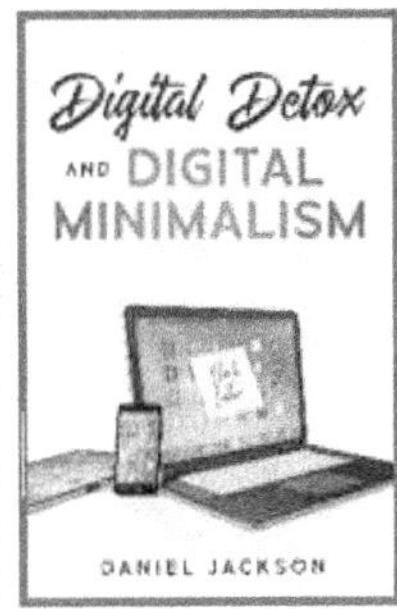

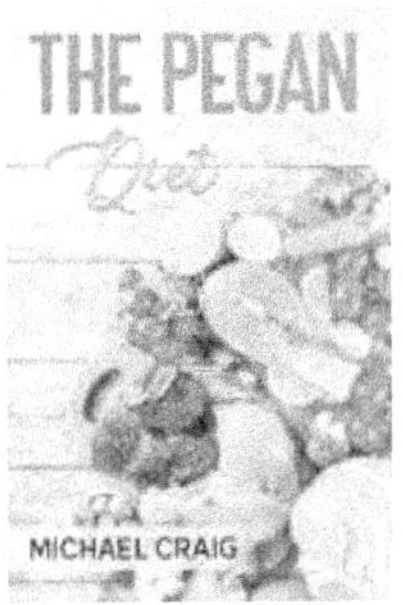

Take a look at more great books available from Rockwood Publishing

… some for FREE!

Just visit the link below:

rockwoodpublishing.co.uk

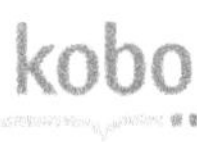

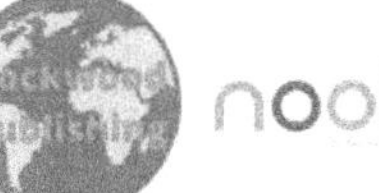

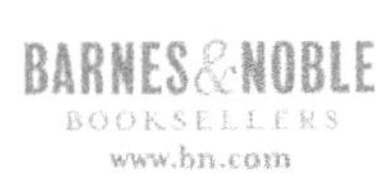

Table of Contents

Honey and Ginger Lemonade

Honey and Vanilla Lemonade

Raw Honey & Lemon Thumbprint Cookies

Q and A

Final Thoughts

Introduction

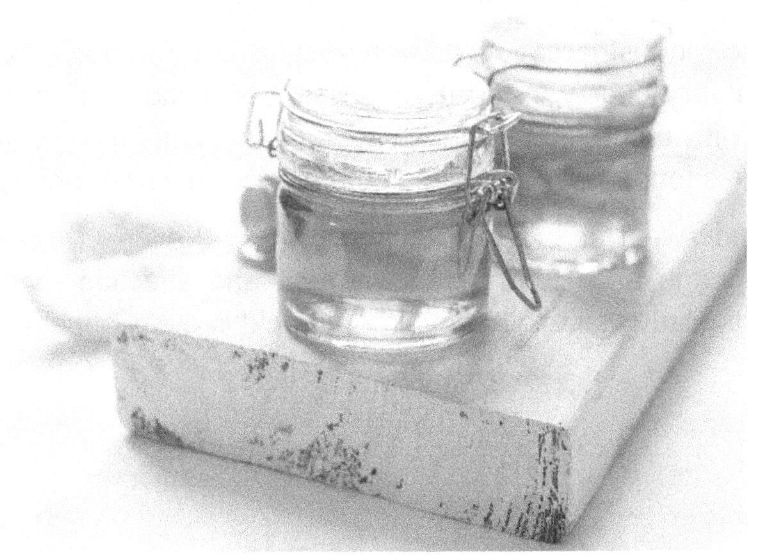

Honey, mentioned as early as Biblical times when God offered freedom to the Pharaoh if he would allow the oppressed people to escape to the land of milk and honey, and, more recently, eight thousand years ago, when a wall painting in Valencia, Spain, depicted figures collecting honeycombs.

Honey appears consistently down the ages as both an immensely desirable food and as a treatment. It was deemed to contain mythical properties and, still, today is valued almost more for its curative properties than as a straightforward delicious food, which it undoubtedly is.

Manuka honey, which originates from New Zealand, is viewed by many to be the Queen amongst honey, and this is because of its amazing nutritional profile.

Since industrialisation and increasing urbanisation, honey can vary hugely in terms of where it is gathered from and how it's processed. Manuka honey has a nutritional content that is four times greater than that of normal flower honey.

From sweet ambrosia to a healing salve, even in modern language as a term of endearment and affection, honey, particularly Manuka honey, is solid gold in every aspect.

Graham Hodson

What Is Manuka Honey?

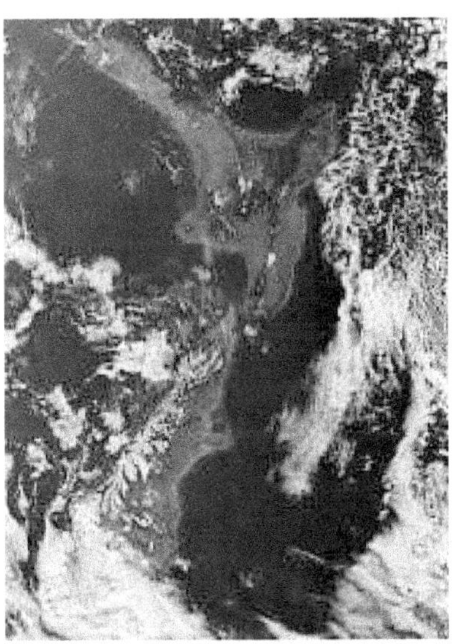

Manuka honey is a monofloral honey produced from the small white flowers of the wild Manuka tree (*Leptospermum scoparium)* which <u>only</u> grows in New Zealand on the North Island. This in itself makes Manuka honey quite unique, but it has acquired a reputation of excellence for one other main reason:

Manuka honey has a nutritional value up to four times greater than that of normal flower honey.

Before discussing the value and benefits of Manuka honey in particular, it is important to understand how honey is harvested and processed in the modern age.

There are several hundred honey varieties available from all across the globe and whilst source is key to your choice of honey, how that honey has been harvested and treated is also integral to what you are buying.

Honey can be supplied in a raw or pasteurised form, filtered or unfiltered, as comb, liquid or in whipped form, and from either a local or an imported source.

As you might imagine, the purest form of honey is the most beneficial as this has not been tampered with and corrupted or devalued, the same as with other food stuffs. So raw honey is better in terms of its nutritional profile than processed honey, and raw honey already has a tremendous reputation for excellent nutritional benefits and as an immune booster.

Raw honey is rich in essential minerals such as copper, iron and magnesium and the B vitamin complex, but Manuka honey is superior even to this.

In 1981, researchers led by Professor Peter Molan based at the University of Waikato in New Zealand realised that Manuka honey has much higher levels of enzymes than normal raw flower honey.

The combined effect of these enzymes is to produce natural hydrogen peroxide which operates as an antibacterial agent similar in strength to either phenol or carbolic acid. This was verified in the Biological Sciences department of the University in their testing.

There are different strains of Manuka honey and the best is rich in the "holy trinity" of hydrogen peroxide, methylglyoxal and dihydroxyacetone, but not all Manuka flowers produce these three components from their nectar.

These three components when present are referred to as the Unique Manuka Factor or UMF, and this has now been formalised as a global standard that assures the user that the Manuka honey in question is of a medicinal quality with antibacterial properties.

Nutritional and Medicinal Benefits of Manuka Honey

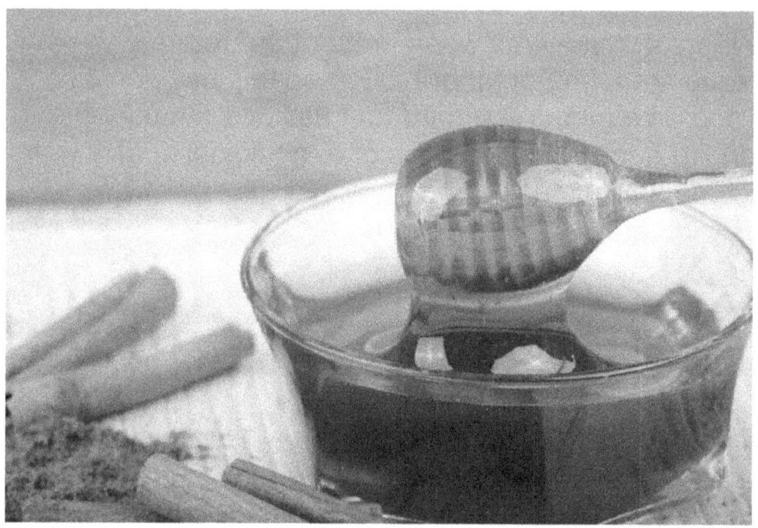

Manuka honey, produced in New Zealand by bees that pollinate the Manuka bush, is one of the most unique and beneficial forms of honey in the world. Here are some of the nutritional elements (in alphabetical order, not in order of concentration levels) that can be found in Manuka honey:-

- Amino acids

- B vitamins (B6, thiamin, niacin, riboflavin, pantothenic acid)

- Calcium

- Copper

- Iron

- Magnesium

- Manganese

- Phosphorus

- Potassium

- Sodium

Manuka honey is known to have natural antibiotic, antiseptic, antioxidant, anti-inflammatory, and antimicrobial qualities, and so its uses for any bacterial issues are well documented. But there are a variety of other illnesses and conditions for which Manuka honey is also appropriate as a treatment and these are the principal ones on the list: -

Acid Reflux and Stomach Acid

Stomach Acid and Acid Reflux are closely related conditions and Manuka honey is a common panacea used to re-balance the digestive system and combat intestinal issues.

IBS and IBD

Irritable Bowel Syndrome or IBS and its close neighbour, Irritable Bowel Disease or IBD, have been shown to respond well when sufferers have taken Manuka honey. Typical symptoms of both IBS and IBD are diarrhoea or conversely constipation, alternating between the two, irregular bowel movement often caused by the swing from diarrhoea to constipation and back again, and chronic abdominal pain.

Some studies have indicated that Manuka honey may be beneficial in treating the symptoms of IBS and IBD although it is not yet clear how this process actually works.

Certainly, in general terms, Manuka honey is well recognised for having anti-inflammatory benefits and inflammation of the intestine and bowel is a common symptom of both these conditions although it is important to remember that IBS and IBD are still different diseases.

In August 2008, the Chandigarh Postgraduate Institute of Medical Education and Research (India) performed a study that focused on the antioxidant effect of Manuka honey and how relevant and helpful this may be to the treatment of IBD.

The study, admittedly on rats, not humans, indicated that levels of intestinal inflammation decreased in those rats which were treated with Manuka honey.

What was also interesting is that the study revealed that the rats which had also suffered oxidative damage also improved following treatment with Manuka honey as the honey improved the antioxidant parameters.

Oxygen is an essential component of our bodily function. During the metabolic processes within the body, molecules of oxygen are subjected to several reactions and in certain circumstances, this can produce an unstable oxygen molecule that is harmful to the human body, particularly the organs and tissues.

These molecules are implicated in the causes of certain diseases and conditions where they are found to have accumulated within the body and amongst these are IBS and IBD.

The researchers found that not only did the Manuka honey have a beneficial effect on inflammation within the gastrointestinal tract, but that oxidative stress, which is a feature of Irritable Bowel Syndrome, also responded favourably to the ingestion of the honey.

Manuka honey was found by researchers to operate through the toll-like receptor pathway. Toll-like receptors or TLRs are a group of proteins that have a key role in the immune system, this is where the cells proliferate and the immune response and inflammation are triggered.

Manuka honey appears to reduce swelling associated with inflammation and also prevents activation of inflammatory cells in the first place, a double-headed benefit as the honey treats both the current condition and also help to protect against future damage.

Acne and Eczema

Countless people have reported that Manuka honey, when applied directly to the skin, can improve both acne and eczema. However, there have been no clinical investigations into these claims thus far.

Because Manuka honey has both healing and antimicrobial properties, it is easy to see why people who suffer from these conditions have applied it to their skin, with beneficial results.

Infections

The anti-microbial properties of Manuka Honey have made it a popular choice in place of, or in addition to, modern antibiotics. Some of the bad boys include Clostridium Difficile, E Coli, Campylobacter, and Enterobacter, some of which are implicated in infections that can pre-herald conditions such as IBS.

These bacteria are susceptible to the anti-microbial effects of Manuka honey and in the modern age, where superbugs such as Methicillin-resistant Staphylococcus Aureus, more commonly known as MRSA, are becoming increasingly resistant to antibiotics, Manuka honey is beginning to present itself as a real and valid alternative for bacterial treatment.

Scientists at the University of Cardiff led by Professor Les Baillie have been conducting research to examine the potential use of Manuka honey in fighting the new generation of hospital superbugs[1].

Professor Baillie, who is from the Welsh School of Pharmacy and Pharmaceutical Sciences, in conjunction with the National Botanic Garden of Wales, has been examining the antibacterial properties of Manuka honey and it is the aim of the team to identify native British plants with similar health benefits, and they are doing this by collecting and analysing honey samples from all over the United Kingdom.

Currently focusing on Welsh honey, the team are determining the DNA profile of the honey with the inclusion of other honey from across the British Isles so as to increase their knowledge base and diversity.

Such is the interest and importance of the scheme that funding has been obtained from the Welsh Government and the European Social Fund as well as the University itself.

Wounds, burns and ulcers

As well as ingesting Manuka, the honey can also be applied topically to the skin and is used to promote the healing of

---

[1]   http://www.cardiff.ac.uk/news/view/56308-honey-needed-for-superbug-fight

wounds and to offer pain relief to patients suffering from burns.

Manuka honey's anti-inflammatory properties provide soothing relief and the antibacterial element can assist in combating infection; for both of these reasons, Manuka honey is also a popular choice in treating ulcers.

Manuka honey's antibacterial components are thought to be due to its high-level osmolarity – the concentration of a solution expressed as the total number of solute particles per litre – of hydrogen peroxide.

The high osmolarity of the honey draws lymph from the wound and the dissolved nutrients contained within the lymph are a source of nutrition for the regeneration of the tissue.

Gingivitis and tooth decay

You wouldn't expect a substance with a naturally sweet content to be the first port of call for decay issues within the mouth, but scientists from the University of Otago's School of Dentistry in New Zealand discovered that a 35% decrease in plaque production could be achieved by sucking or chewing on a product which contained Manuka honey. This process also reduced bleeding in those patients who also suffered from Gingivitis.

Immunity issues and sore throats

The Journal of Leukocyte Biology published data in 2007 which reviewed the composition of Manuka honey which stated that "A5.8-kDa component of Manuka honey stimulates immune cells via TLR4".

More information appeared in the public domain in 2011 which supports the use of Manuka honey for sore throats as it inhibits the growth of the Streptococcus bacteria.

It has long been recognised that a spoonful of honey soothes a sore throat with its anti-inflammatory and lubricant elements but now it seems that Manuka honey will also actually help fight the harmful bacteria that cause the issue in the first place.

Sinusitis and other allergies

Honey has long been recognised as a suitable relief for allergy sufferers because of its anti-inflammatory and antioxidant properties.

Standard prescription and over the counter remedies such as antihistamines and steroids can cause side effects and increasingly, people are looking outside the standard healthcare range for alternative remedies.

There is currently no scientific data to support the use of any honey as a treatment to combat the misery-inducing symptoms of seasonal allergies and sinusitis, but there is plenty of anecdotal evidence.

Honey and Manuka honey contains the same range of pollen spores that cause so much suffering to those individuals who are seasonally sensitive.

The theory is that by introducing these agents to the body in small and ever-increasing quantities, the body's immune system alters its response over time and so when the real article arrives in the atmosphere in abundance, the body simply does not react or certainly does not react as strongly because the immune system is already familiar with the substances.

This is nature's perfect immunotherapy.

Students at the Xavier University in New Orleans conducted an informal study across a range of allergy sufferers in an attempt to calculate the effect or otherwise, that honey had on them.

Whilst this was not an official, regulated study, the results were positive with reports that symptoms in both seasonal allergy sufferers and the group who suffered year-round with symptoms were both reduced and improved. [2]

---

[2] Cochran, Brittany. "Honey: A sweet relief?" Xavier University. October 23, 2003.

Health and Beauty - the Role of Manuka Honey

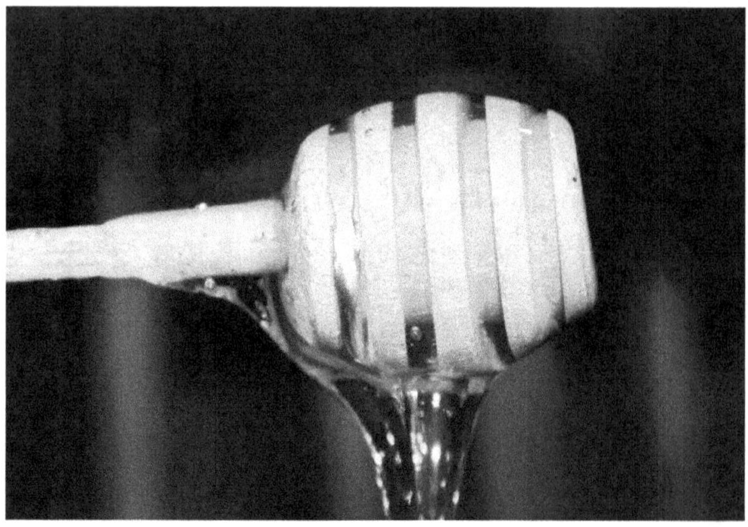

The beneficial properties of Manuka honey for health and beauty have long been known through the ages.

Manuka honey has the effect of an elixir and was used by ancient peoples as a gift to accompany the dead into the afterlife and as offering the God of Fertility in ancient Egypt.

The Indians believed that honey had healing and also spiritual powers and in Hinduism, it is still one of the five elixirs of immortality, whilst in the Jewish faith, it is a symbol of New Year and renewal.

Honey is referenced in the New Testament as a source of sustenance and in Islam, the Prophet Mohammad describes honey as a healthy and nutritious food and as a source of healing.

As a beauty tool, Manuka honey can be used in a number of different ways to cleanse, improve both skin tone and texture and promote youthful vigour and energy.

There are myriad products available that contain Manuka honey or you could simply make your own honey. Manuka honey makes a perfect face wash or shampoo; you can just add it to your usual product or use it on its own.

Inner health is just as important as outer and combining honey with a homemade health drink, or just adding a little to some hot water, means that you can harness the cleansing and revitalizing potency of Manuka honey both inside your body as well as outside.

Sleep has long been recognised as a key component in human health. Manuka honey can help promote deep and restful sleep, acting on your body whilst it is at rest.

Manuka honey helps the body to release melatonin which is a hormone made by the pineal gland in the brain. Melatonin is essential for the control of the sleeping and waking cycles and a lack of it can cause disturbed sleep patterns with all the associated health issues that can accompany poor nighttime rest.

Manuka honey added to some warm milk at bedtime can help promote the release of melatonin and assist with deep and restful sleep.

The Role of Manuka Honey in Treating Animals

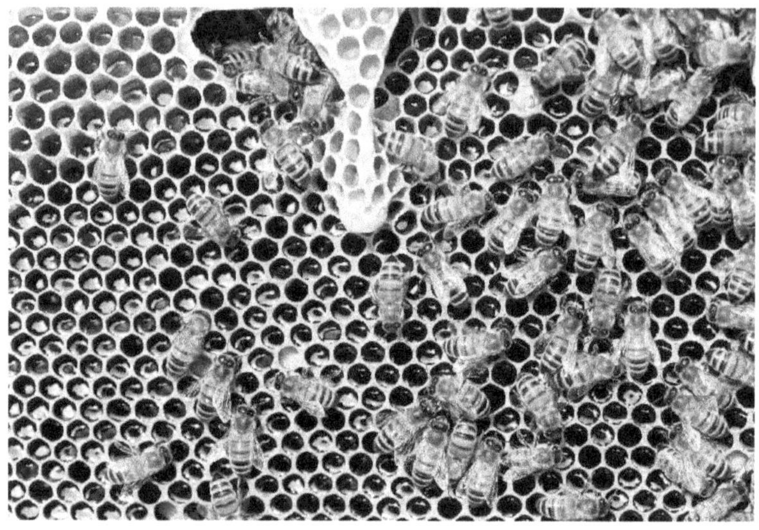

Manuka honey has been recognised as an efficient and effective product to treat wounds and skin issues, even burns, in both small and large animals.

Veterinary Surgeon Louise O' Dwyer discusses the important influence of Manuka honey in the Veterinary Ireland Journal[3] in which she states that the specific qualities of honey in the healing process were, "decreased inflammatory oedema, the attraction of macrophages to further cleanse the wound, accelerated sloughing of devitalised tissue, provision of a local cellular energy source,

---

[3] http://www.veterinaryirelandjournal.com/images/nurse_sep_2016.pdf

and formation of a protective layer of protein over the wound and a healthy granulation bed."

The veterinary profession has perhaps been slower than pet owners to appreciate the value of Manuka honey as a treatment, principally because vets are scientists, so are only interested in treatments with proven, scientific efficacy.

Animal owners have been using Manuka honey for years and with the advent of social media and online forums, the exchange of advice and information has become ever easier.

Manuka Honey Products

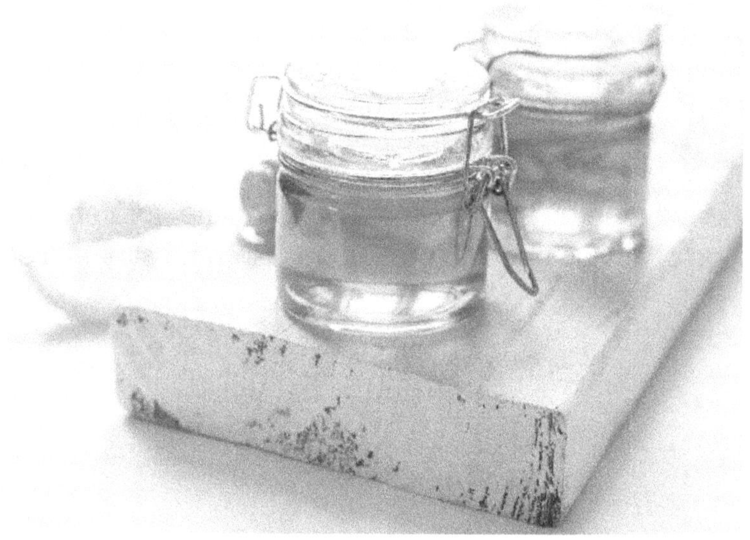

The healthcare benefits of Manuka honey are no secret and so there is a huge range of products on the market which contain this Queen of Honeys.

Celebrity endorsement of Manuka honey abounds; the American actress, singer and model Scarlett Johansson uses Manuka honey as a face mask to improve the radiance of her skin and Czech supermodel and television host, Petra Nemcova, uses Manuka honey as a facial cleanser.

She bases her claim to flawless skin on the honey stating that it removes impurities and leaves her with a glow that is only too evident.

Katherine Jenkins, the opera singer, who might be forgiven for using Manuka honey on her face, so beautiful is her skin, actually uses it to protect and enhance her most famous asset – her voice. Katherine drinks Manuka honey in hot water regularly to help keep her performance tip-top.

Catherine Zeta-Jones, Hollywood superstar, does use Manuka honey on her skin, a mix of salt and Manuka honey providing the perfect detoxifying scrub for her skin.

Lizzie Jagger, the famous model and probably more famously daughter of Rolling Stone, Mick Jagger, uses a Manuka honey not only as a lip balm to protect her lips and moisturise them, but also as a barrier repellent against germs.

Skincare

Manuka honey is used extensively in a range of different skincare treatments. The list below is by no means exhaustive:-

- Moisturising day creams for the face

- Intensive nourishing night-time creams

- Facial masks for repair and rejuvenation

- Facial scrubs where Manuka honey is combined with an exfoliant such as bamboo particles

- Anti-ageing serums

- Healing creams for irritated, sunburnt or inflamed skin

- Cream treatments for facial acne

- Lip balms and sun salve

Joint Care

Manuka honey has been used in balms to relieve sore muscles and joints due to its anti-inflammatory and soothing properties.

Graham Hodson

Where to Buy Manuka Honey

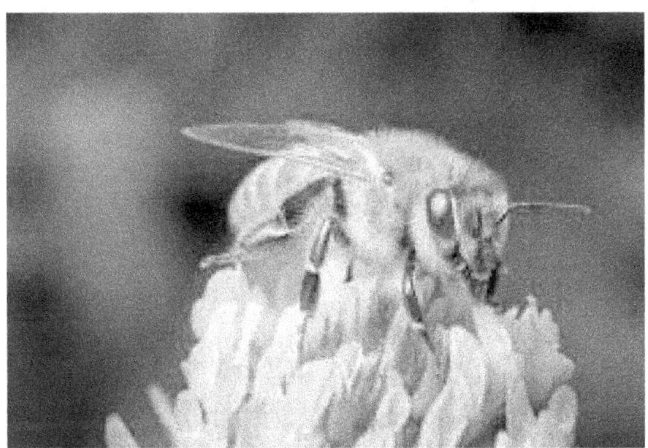

As imitation is the sincerest form of flattery, you can imagine that the market is full of fake Manuka products which make all sorts of health claims and which are not the real deal.

Official figures in the Grocer magazine state that there are around 10,000 tons of Manuka honey sold each year, but apparently, only 1,700 tons of the genuine article is actually produced, so a good number of manufacturers are being somewhat less than honest!

So, the simplest and most effective advice in connection with where to buy Manuka honey is from **only the most reputable, established online or high street stores.**

When going the online route, I highly recommend: -

If you live in the USA: -

manukahoneyusa.com

If you live in the UK: -

manukahoney.co.uk

There are others, of course, and if you live anywhere else in the world there will be reputable sellers in your country also, but I have dealt with the two companies stated above so can personally vouch for their professionalism and quality of product and service.

You must also look for a high UMF (Unique Manuka Factor) number or MGO (methylglyoxal) number if you are to use the honey medicinally.

All honey has some degree of antibacterial activity because of the naturally occurring hydrogen peroxide within the honey.

What makes Manuka honey so special is that it can have what's called "non-peroxide activity or NPA" as well as the antibacterial properties from the hydrogen peroxide.

However, not all Manuka honey has NPA activity.

As already stated, all honey has some degree of an anti-bacterial action, but it's been found that Manuka honey's anti-microbial activity is a lot more potent than normal honey.

In normal honey, the hydrogen peroxide breaks down resulting in the anti-bacterial activity being lost. Manuka honey, on the other hand, contains methylglyoxal, which continues to be active after the hydrogen peroxide is lost.

This is the non-peroxide activity to which was previously referred.

Personally, I would ALWAYS choose to use the UMF system of classification as it is an internationally recognised trademark that can <u>only</u> be used by licensed Manuka honey producers exclusively from New Zealand who produce natural, unmodified, unrefined, pure Manuka honey.

There are several 'fake' rating systems used by honey manufacturing companies in an attempt to disguise lower-grade honey.

Avoid any honey that doesn't specify either its UMF or MGO content as it is highly unlikely to be genuine Manuka honey.

The only way a Manuka honey can gain the UMF grading is to pass independent tests.

Equivalent UMF to MGO table for easy reference: -

UMF	MGO (mg/kg)
5+	83
10+	263
12+	356
15+	514
18+	696
20+	829

It is always worth considering two important factors when looking at the strength of Manuka honey: -

1. A high strength Manuka honey can be used for ALL purposes, medicinal or non-medicinal, but a low strength one cannot be used for medicinal purposes.

2. If the honey is to be used for helping any digestive issues, then its strength will be diluted by the very act of swallowing and mixing it with saliva and other digestive juices. In this case, it's best to opt for a honey of higher strength in order to help counter this unavoidable dilution.

How to Take Manuka Honey

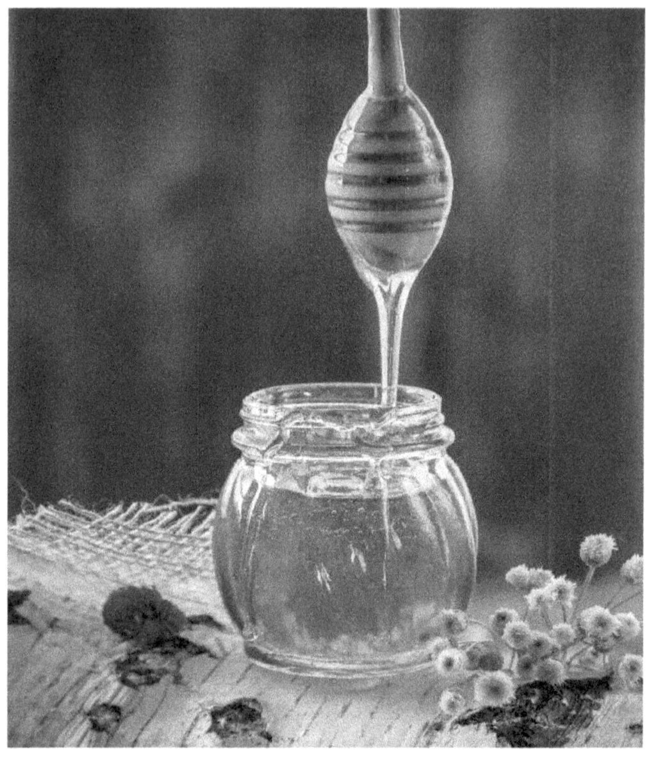

Some people react to honey and it is possible to be allergic to it, so it is recommended that a patch test is undertaken to ensure that Manuka honey is safe to consume.

Manuka honey is not recommended for use in babies below the age of twelve months as there can be a risk of infant botulism poisoning due to the bacteria contained within it. Current medical advice, therefore, is to avoid giving even the tiniest quantity of honey to an infant below the age of twelve months.[4]

Because of the increased sugar levels in Manuka and indeed in any honey, those people who suffer from diabetes should maintain a close eye on their blood sugar levels when consuming Manuka honey.

It is not the purpose of this article to advise as to the use of Manuka honey in the first place - that is entirely at the reader's discretion - nor is it intended to offer any guidance as to dosage if you do decide to use it.

With the above precautions in mind, it is strongly advised that you use/take Manuka honey <u>exactly</u> as directed on the label of the bottle or container or follow the guidance offered in the manufacturer's guideline leaflet.

---

[4]   http://www.mayoclinic.org/healthy-lifestyle/infant-and-toddler-health/expert-answers/infant-botulism/faq-20058477

Recipes

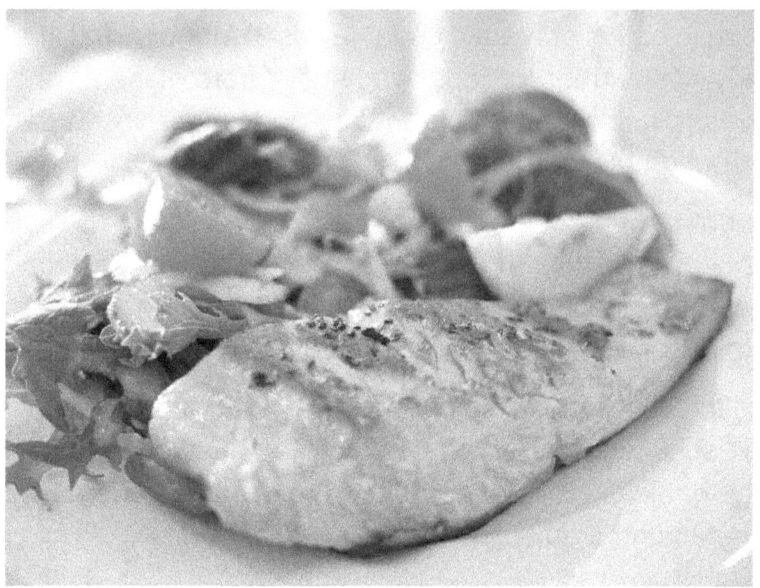

So, we've firmly established that Manuka honey is incredible stuff!

It tastes amazing and is so good for us that it truly deserves the sub-heading of this book... One of Nature's Miracles.

Obviously, its uses are manyfold, from the elaborate to the every day spreading on hot toast, but there are just so many amazing recipes that can incorporate Manuka honey and the following are just the "tip of the iceberg" and intended not only for your delight, but also to act as inspiration for further experimentation.

Who knows what culinary masterpiece you could come up with!

The following recipes are, with very kind permission, taken from the fabulous website: -

manukahoneyusa.com

It's a truly fabulous site with anything and everything to do with manuka honey and I can recommend it wholeheartedly.

My sincere thanks to them for their generous permission to include these awesome recipes.

Raw Honey and Garlic Green Beans

Ingredients:

- Fresh green beans (recipe is for roughly 50 fresh beans), ends cut
- 2 tablespoons olive oil
- 1 clove fresh garlic, peeled, crushed, and minced
- 2 tablespoons raw honey
- Red paper flakes (to taste – optional)
- Salt and pepper, to taste

Directions:

1. Heat large skillet over medium heat
2. When the pan is warmed, add olive oil and heat
3. After the olive oil has been heated, add garlic to flavour
4. Add green beans to the mix and toss to ensure beans are completely covered in olive oil
5. Continue to cook green beans, tossing occasionally, for about five minutes
6. Green beans should start to lightly brown on all sides before the next step
7. Add honey to the pan and toss again to ensure there is some honey on all of the beans

8. Cook for an additional 30 seconds or so to ensure the honey has been warmed

9. Just before removing, add salt and pepper to taste

10. Remove beans and place in serving dish or on plates

11. If desired, lightly sprinkle the beans with chilli pepper flakes

Honey Garlic Chicken

Ingredients:

- 2 pounds chicken breast, skinned, cut into chunks
- 2 tablespoons olive or coconut oil
- 3 minces garlic gloves
- ¾ teaspoon dried basil
- 1/3 cup soy sauce
- 1/3 cup ketchup
- ¼ cup raw honey
- 1/8 teaspoon red pepper flakes
- ½ cup bourbon (optional if you want to give the dish a bit more of a punch)

Directions:

1. In a large sauté pan, heat oil, then add chicken cubes to sear off before placing in a slow cooker.
2. In a small bowl, combine basil, garlic, soy sauce, ketchup, raw honey, and bourbon (if used).
3. Add seared chicken to crockpot, then pour sauce over top and combine all ingredients.
4. Put the slow cooker on low setting, cover, and allow to cook.

I like to let the dish simmer overnight, but it will be ready to go in about four or five hours. If you are going to let it simmer overnight, you can add some chicken stock to the crockpot to ensure it will not reduce down too much overnight.

The dish can be served over rice or is delicious enough all on its own.

<u>Banana, Nut, and Manuka Honey Cupcakes</u>

Ingredients:

Cupcakes:

- 2 cups of whole wheat flour
- 1 teaspoon of baking powder
- 1 teaspoon of baking soda
- 1/4 teaspoon of ground cinnamon
- Pinch of salt
- 4 large bananas (preferably ripe)
- 1/4 cup of Manuka honey
- 1/4 cup of brown sugar
- 1 tablespoon of melted coconut oil
- 1 teaspoon of vanilla
- 1 egg
- 2 tablespoons of chopped walnuts
- 1/4 cup of smooth peanut butter
- 1/2 cup of milk

Icing:

- 1/4 cup of peanut butter
- 1 cup of cream cheese
- 1-2 tablespoons of cream
- 1 cup of powdered sugar
- 1 teaspoon of vanilla

Directions:

1. To begin, preheat your oven to 350 degrees Fahrenheit on the Bake setting. Spray a muffin tray with cooking spray or line with paper cups.

2. Peel the bananas, and then start mashing them with a fork until a smooth texture forms.

3. Place the mashed bananas into a mixer before adding the Manuka honey, the brown sugar, the melted coconut oil, the vanilla, and the egg. Mix the ingredients well. Add the smooth peanut butter to the bunch, beating until well incorporated.

4. In a separate mixing bowl, mix the flour, the baking powder, the baking soda, the ground cinnamon, and the salt. Add this dry mixture to the wet mixture along with the milk and the walnuts, mixing thoroughly.

5. Spoon the mixture into the muffin tray, and then bake for roughly 20 minutes or till a toothpick or fork comes up clean.

6. While the cupcakes are cooling, start making the icing. Add the peanut butter, cream cheese, powdered sugar, cream, and vanilla to an available mixing bowl. Once the cupcakes are ready, frost them with your peanut butter icing.

7. Serve the cupcakes immediately or at your discretion afterwards. These cupcakes should store well for at least a week in your fridge.

<u>Manuka Honey Pizza Dough</u>

<u>*Total Prep/Cook Time*</u>*: 30 min.*

<u>*Servings*</u>*: Eight.*

Ingredients:

- 1 package of dry yeast, quick rise
- 1 cup of lukewarm water
- 1 tablespoon of Manuka honey
- 2 tablespoons of olive, vegetable, or canola oil
- 2½ cups of whole wheat flour, white
- ½ teaspoon of onion powder
- ½ teaspoon of garlic powder

Directions:

1. To begin, mix the yeast and the lukewarm water in a large glass bowl. From there, add the Manuka honey, the oil, the whole wheat flour, the onion powder, and the garlic powder.

2. If you don't have a standing mixer, grease your hands lightly to prep them for non-stick mixing, and then mix everything well. <u>Note</u>: If you do have a standing mixer, be sure to lightly grease the bowl first before mixing any ingredients.

3. Let the dough sit in the bowl for between five and ten minutes while covered by a damp towel.

4. Roll the pizza dough out to a suitable thickness, one that ideally fits an 18 x 13-inch half-sheet pan. Flatten the dough on the pan after lightly greasing the pan beforehand.

5. Bake the dough in your oven at 450 degrees Fahrenheit for around five minutes. Remove the dough from the oven, add your preferred toppings, and then bake the pizza for roughly ten extra minutes.

6. This recipe calls for all-purpose white flour or whole wheat white flour. If you want to use brown whole wheat flour instead, mix 1¼ cups of brown whole grain flour and 1¼ cups of white flour.

Homemade Manuka Honey Fig Bars

Ingredients:

Filling:

- 2 cups of dried figs
- 1/4 cup of Manuka honey
- 3/4 cup of cold water
- 1 tablespoon of orange zest
- 1/2 teaspoon of salt

Cookie:

- 1 cup of oats
- 2 cups of oat flour
- 1/2 cup of chopped walnuts
- 1 teaspoon of baking soda
- 1 tablespoon of grounded chia seeds
- 2 teaspoons of cinnamon
- 1/3 cup of Manuka honey
- 1/2 cup of unsweetened applesauce
- 2 teaspoons of vanilla extract
- 1/2 cup of olive oil

Directions:

1. To begin, remove the stems of the dried figs, and then place the figs into a saucepan with your cold water. Let them soak for about 15 minutes.

2. For the filling, mix in the Manuka honey, the salt, and the orange zest before bringing to boil, reducing to simmer, and then cooking for about 30 minutes. After that, set to the side to cool down for around 15 minutes, and then puree everything to a paste using a blender or food processor.

3. After lining parchment paper along a 9in by 9in baking dish, preheat your oven to 350 degrees Fahrenheit. Combine the oats, the oat flour, the walnuts, the baking soda, the chia seeds, and the cinnamon in a large bowl before setting it aside.

4. In another large bowl, mix the Manuka honey, the vanilla extract, the applesauce, and the olive oil, stirring.

5. Add your dry mixture to your wet mixture, stirring until it's just combined. Put half the dough in the baking dish, pressing firmly for the base layer. Note: The dough is sticky, so using parchment paper to press it down should keep the dough from getting stuck on your hands. Smearing your hands with olive oil should also keep the dough off your hands.

6. Scoop the fig filling out from your food processor, and then lay it thinly on your base cookie layer and press till a smooth second layer has formed.

7. Spoon the remaining oat batter onto the fig filling and smooth it down evenly. From there, bake the fig bars for around 30 minutes or until they've developed a golden-brown colour.

8. Remove the fig bars from your oven and let them cool for a couple of hours. <u>Note</u>: This ensures your fig bars will hold together correctly. Store them inside a sealed, airtight container for as much as three days.

Graham Hodson

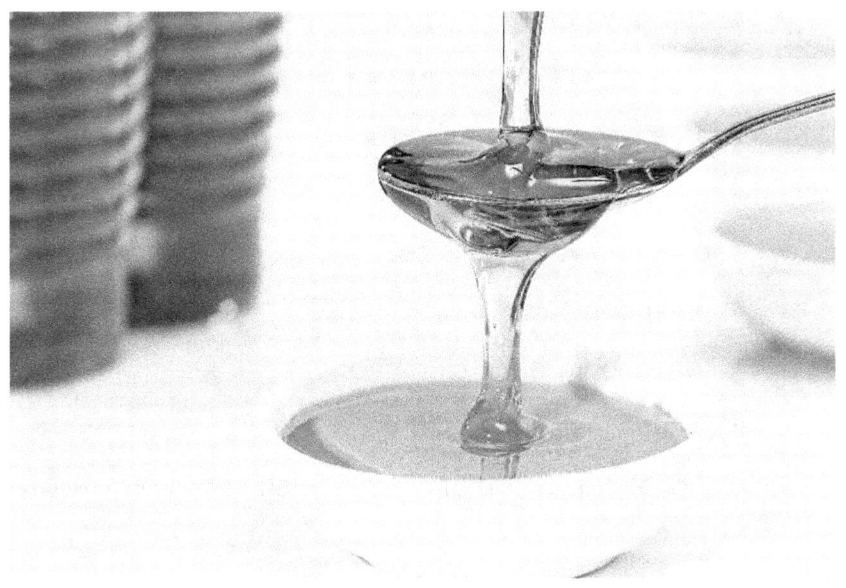

39

Honey Banana Bread

Ingredients:

- 1/3 cup coconut oil
- ½ cup raw honey
- 2 eggs
- 2 large bananas (mashed)
- 1 teaspoon baking soda
- 1 teaspoon vanilla extract
- ½ teaspoon salt
- ½ teaspoon ground cinnamon
- 1 ¾ cup whole wheat flour
- Optional: half a cup of chocolate chips

Directions:

1. Preheat oven to 325 degrees Fahrenheit.
2. While the oven is warming up, grease up a 9*5 loaf pan.
3. In a large mixing bowl, combine oil and honey and whisk together.
4. When those ingredients are fully integrated, add eggs, bananas, and milk.
5. Continue to whisk together until well combined.

6. Add baking soda, vanilla, salt, and cinnamon, and whisk until combined.

7. With a large wooden spoon or spatula, fold in flour (mixture can be a little lumpy).

8. If you are adding chocolate chips or nuts, fold in these ingredients now as well.

9. Once the batter is ready, pour into a loaf pan.

10. For a "chef" effect, take a little more cinnamon and sprinkle a line of it right down the middle of the batter, then use a knife to create a pattern with the cinnamon.

11. Place loaf pan in the oven and bake for 55-60 minutes.

12. You can start checking the bread at 55 minutes with a toothpick (it should come out of the batter clean).

13. Remove the bread from the oven and allow it to cool in the loaf pan for about 10 minutes, then transfer to a wire rack to cool for an additional 20 minutes before serving.

This bread is going to be super-moist and tastes better warm than cold.

Peanut Butter and Raw Honey Fudge

Ingredients:

- 1 cup granulated sugar
- ¼ cup almond milk
- 1C natural creamy peanut butter
- 1 tablespoon raw honey (use either Manuka or Pohutukawa honey)
- 5 teaspoon vanilla extract

Directions:

1. Spray an 8 x 8 baking pan or dish with coconut oil (this is going to add a little extra flavour to the fudge as well (you can substitute olive oil if you prefer)
2. In a small pot, add sugar and milk over high heat
3. Stir ingredients to combine and bring to a boil
4. Continue to stir the mixture while it boils and cook for an additional three minutes
5. After three minutes, turn off the flame, then gradually add peanut butter to the mix
6. Once the peanut butter is added and combined, add honey, continuing to stir to ensure all ingredients are thoroughly combined

7. Add vanilla extract and stir again to ensure ingredients are combined

8. Pour mixture into baking dish and refrigerate for a minimum of six hours

9. For best results, allow the mixture to remain refrigerated overnight

Now all you need to do is cut it into pieces and share... *or not!*

Homemade Manuka Honey Ice Cream

Ingredients:

- 2 cans Thai coconut milk (about 14oz each)
- 3 ounces Manuka honey (1/4 cup and two tablespoons)
- ½ teaspoon xanthan gum (can substitute 1 tablespoon arrowroot powder)
- 1 tablespoon vanilla extract
- Pinch of sea salt

Directions:

1. Using a blender, combine all ingredients
2. Allow mixture to cool in the fridge overnight
3. Using an ice cream machine, process the mixture according to the manufacturer's instructions.
4. Once the ice cream is processed, divide into equal portions in individual containers
5. Cover and freeze until you are ready to eat (we recommend freezing ice cream for at least four hours before serving)
6. When ready to serve, drizzle the ice cream with honey for an additional pop

7. Per our picture, one service suggestion is to serve the ice cream over waffles or a warmed piece of pie or cake

You can play around with this recipe to change the flavours. Blueberries, strawberries, peaches, or nuts can create a completely different taste of ice cream.

Slow Cooked Honey Baked Beans

Ingredients:

- ½ lb dried Great Northern Beans (rinsed)
- 1 medium onion (sliced)
- 4 cups water
- ¼ cup Manuka honey (can substitute Blue Borage honey)
- 4 cloves garlic (minced)
- 2 tablespoons tomato paste
- 2 tablespoons olive oil
- 1 ½ teaspoons salt
- 1 teaspoon mashed chipotle chilies in adobo sauce

Directions:

1. Place dried beans in a medium-sized saucepan. Add water to the beans until they are covered with water. Bring beans to a boil then reduce heat until the beans are simmering. Cook beans in the simmering water for 30 minutes. Remove saucepan from the stove and drain beans from water. Set aside.

2. Move the oven rack to the centre of the oven. Preheat the oven to 325 degrees Fahrenheit.

3. In an oven-proof, 2.5-quart Dutch oven, heat oil over medium-high heat on the stovetop. Add sliced onion and cook until the onion is lightly browned about 4 to

5 minutes. Add tomato paste, garlic, and chipotle pepper. Mix well. Then add beans, water, honey, and salt. Stir until the mixture is well combined.

4. Bring the contents of the Dutch oven to boil over the burner on the stovetop. Cover the Dutch oven with a snug-fitting lid and move to the preheated oven on the centre rack.

5. Bake in the oven until the beans are tender, approximately 3 to 4 hours making sure to stir every hour and add water as needed to keep the beans covered with a "soupy" consistency.

6. Remove from the oven and allow to cool slightly. Serve alongside your favourite main dish and enjoy!

Honey and Ginger Lemonade

Ingredients:

- 6 cups water
- 1 ½ cups of lemon juice (fresh squeezed)
- 1 cup Manuka honey
- 1/3 cup sliced ginger
- Ice cubes

Directions:

1. In a medium saucepan, bring 2 cups of water, honey and sliced ginger to a boil.
2. Remove saucepan from heat and allow honey and ginger to steep for 10 minutes.
3. Strain ginger chunks from water and refrigerate water until cold.
4. In a large pitcher, combine 4 cups cold water, honey/ginger mixture and lemon juice until well combined.
5. Place ice cubes into serving glasses.

Pour lemonade over ice and enjoy!

Honey and Vanilla Lemonade

Ingredients:

- 2 ½ cups lemon juice (freshly squeezed)
- 2 cups water
- 2 cups sugar
- ½ cup Manuka honey
- One vanilla bean
- Lemon wheels for garnish

Directions:

1. Combine 2 cups water, sugar and honey in a large saucepan and cook over medium-high heat.

2. Cut the vanilla bean in half lengthwise. Using the back side of the knife, scrape the interior vanilla seeds from the outer skin. Add the vanilla seeds and the outer skin to the saucepan.

3. Bring the honey and vanilla mixture to a boil, cooking for 5 to 6 minutes. Remove the saucepan from the heat and allow it to cool to room temperature.

4. Add the lemon juice to a large pitcher. Holding a strainer over the top of the pitcher, pour the honey and vanilla mixture into the pitcher, straining out the outer skin of the vanilla bean and other large particles.

5. Add cold water to the pitcher until the amount of liquid equals one gallon. Stir lemonade well.

6. Place ice cubes into serving glasses.

Pour lemonade over ice, garnish with a lemon wheel and enjoy!

Graham Hodson

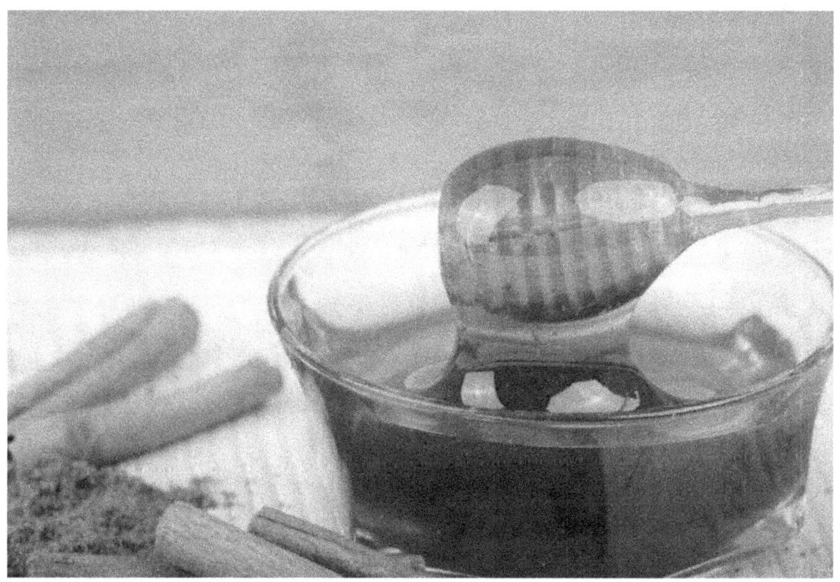

Raw Honey & Lemon Thumbprint Cookies

Ingredients:

- 1½ cups of almond flour
- Zest from 1 lemon, finely grated
- ⅛ teaspoon of fine salt
- ¼ cup of raw honey
- ¼ cup of tahini
- ½ teaspoon of vanilla extract
- 1 teaspoon of olive oil
- 16 chocolate chips or whole almonds (optional)

Directions:

Total Time: 20 min.

Prep Time: 10 min.

Cook Time: 10 min.

Servings: 16 cookies.

1. Preheat your oven to 350 degrees Fahrenheit on the Bake setting. Then, line parchment paper on a baking sheet, preferably one that is rimmed.

2. Using a large bowl, mix the flour, salt, and lemon zest. In another smaller bowl, whisk the tahini, the raw honey, the vanilla, and the olive oil together.

3. Pour your wet ingredients in with your dry ingredients, stirring well until everything has blended. Using your hands, roll the dough until it is in a large ball.

4. Start pinching off pieces of dough roughly one tablespoon in size, rolling them into small balls using your palms.

5. Place the small dough balls on the baking sheet, using up all your dough and putting about one or two inches of space between them. You should have about 16 balls of dough.

6. Press one of your pinkie fingers gently into the middle of every dough ball in order to flatten the cookies slightly until they are each about three-quarters of an inch thick. You can press either a chocolate chip or an almond into each cookie's centre if you prefer.

7. Bake the cookies until their edges have developed a slight brown colour, which should take between 10 and 12 minutes. Once they've finished baking, move the cookies onto a ready wire rack or a sheet of wax paper to cool.

8. You can enjoy the cookies now, store them at room temp in an airtight container for a maximum of two weeks, or freeze them for a max of three months.

Q and A

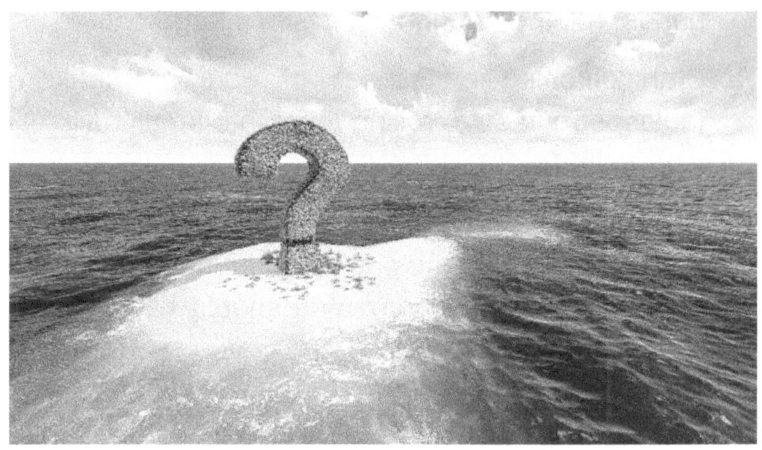

What does Manuka honey TASTE like?

Taste is very subjective and, pun intended, a matter of taste, but a lot of people say that it's got a slightly nutty and herbal aroma which obviously influences how people perceive the nonetheless sweet taste.

Some people also say that the higher the UMF number, the more distinctive the taste.

Where does Manuka honey come from?

(Before I answer this, I ask you to refer to the next question below.)

New Zealand.

It's made by the bees that pollinate the native Manuka flower of New Zealand.

What's this "dispute" I've read about between Australia and New Zealand over the use of the word Manuka?

Take a deep breath…

Manuka honey is produced by bees feeding on the pollen of the *Leptospermum scoparium* plant. Although the plant <u>is</u> grown in areas outside New Zealand, it's known by different names in those parts. It's known as "manuka" in New Zealand, and "tea tree" in Australia.

Therefore, it is logically accepted that the term 'manuka' is seen as a way of differentiating and specifying the plant variety grown only in New Zealand.

However, Australian honey producers claim that the plant (*Leptospermum scoparium)* actually originated in Tasmania (an Australian state south of the mainland) and, over time, dispersed to New Zealand.

In response, New Zealanders claim that "manuka" is a native Maori word and, as such, Australian manufacturers have no right to use it because it implies (some might cynically say deliberately) that the honey comes from New Zealand.

Are you still following this?!

In a counter-response, Australian manufacturers claim that the Maori word for manuka is actually "mānuka" with an inflexion over the 'a', and that they're not trying to claim the Maori name, but merely asserting usage rights to the word manuka, which is, in fact, the universal English interpretation, and, in their opinion, seeing as also how the plant allegedly originated in Australia, that they have very strong and legitimate claims to rightfully use the word manuka.

Phew!

What do DHA and MGO mean?

Nectar from the Mānuka bush contains a substance called Dihydroxyacetone (DHA) which the bees, in turn, convert into methylglyoxal (MGO). It is this compound that has antimicrobial properties.

What is meant by "The Official UMF Release Certificate"?

This presents the test results for all four manuka markers, namely Leptosperin, Methylglyoxal, DHA, and HMF. This must be present on every jar of genuine Manuka honey.

Why is it relatively expensive when compared to other honies?

Because it comes from the somewhat scarce Manuka flower which not only is a natural resource specifically found in New Zealand, but also only flowers for 2 – 6 weeks per year. Add to that the fact that the Manuka flower is particularly sensitive to adverse weather conditions and that some of the hives in which it is produced are incredibly remote and inaccessible and, therefore, very difficult to harvest, it's easy to see why it can be quite expensive.

What's the guarantee that if it says Manuka honey on the jar that it's genuine Manuka honey in the jar?

Good question. Nearly 80% of honey sold as Manuka is fake. New Zealand, the sole point of origin, only produced 1,700 tons of Manuka honey in 2014, but somehow 10,000 tons of it were sold worldwide!

So how do I know if I'm buying "the real deal"?

It can get a little complicated, but here's a "checklist" to help you to be sure that you're spending your hard-earned cash on the genuine article: -

- It has the quality trademark of UMF clearly stated on the front label of the jar

- The honey is genuinely <u>produced</u> in New Zealand

- It is put into jars <u>and</u> labelled on-site in New Zealand

- It comes from a New Zealand based company with an authorised license to use and trade with the quality trademark UMF

- Vitally, it has the UMF Licensee's <u>brand name</u> and <u>licence number</u> on the label

- A rating number <u>with</u> the trademark UMF. Just a number without the UMF is not acceptable

- It must be verified by the Official UMF Release Certificate. This shows the test results for the corresponding batch number shown on the label (see questions above) and is a document that is issued only to UMF-labelled honey that passes all the necessary test criteria.

Are the bees that collect the pollen special manuka bees?

No, they are ordinary European honey bees, brought over to New Zealand in the late 1830s because native bees were not suitable for honey production.

Are the bees OK if we take all their honey?

This is one of my favourite questions because it's so warm-hearted and thoughtful... AND I used to wonder exactly the same thing!

Bees make between two and three times the amount of honey they need as food to survive, so there's plenty to go around. The beekeepers are passionate about their job and lovingly look after the bees.

Final Thoughts

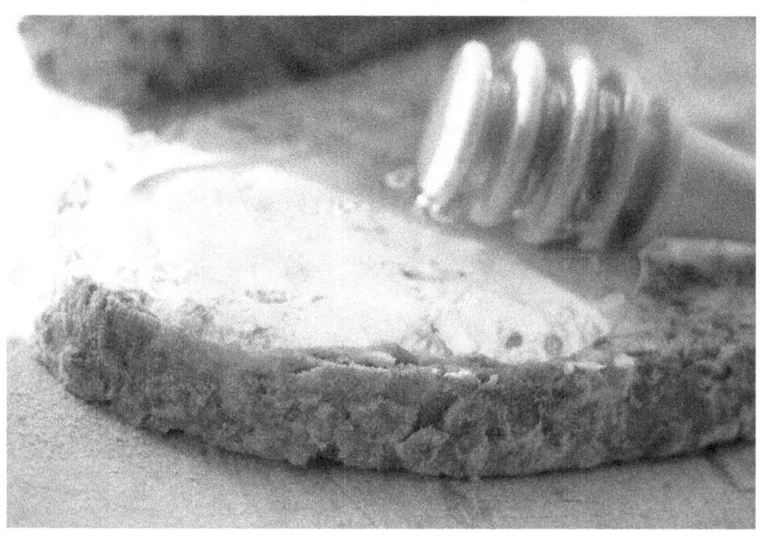

So, there you have it.

A whistle-stop tour of the world of Manuka honey, and what a tasty, healthy world it is too!

It's bizarre to realise that the delicate flowers of the manuka bush and the little honey bees that are attracted to them are the foundation and driving force behind a multi-billion-dollar global industry that provides untold unique health benefits to millions of users worldwide.

I sincerely hope that you enjoyed reading this eBook and that you've gained a greater understanding and appreciation of the power and importance of Manuka honey.

It really is "wonder-stuff" with a myriad of uses…

a veritable powerhouse of nutrition…

and is indeed…

one of nature's miracles!

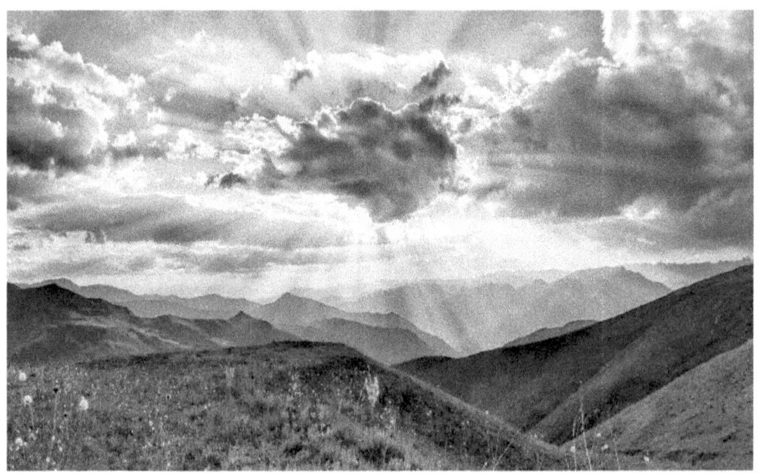

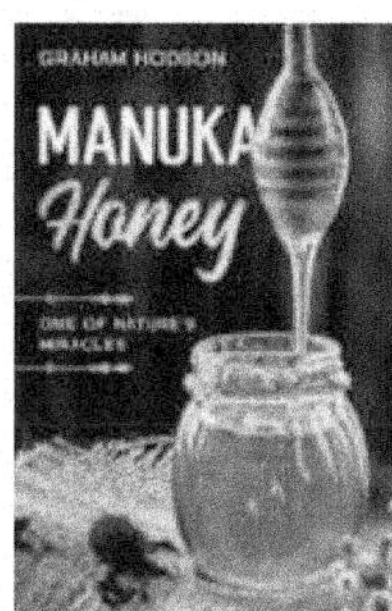

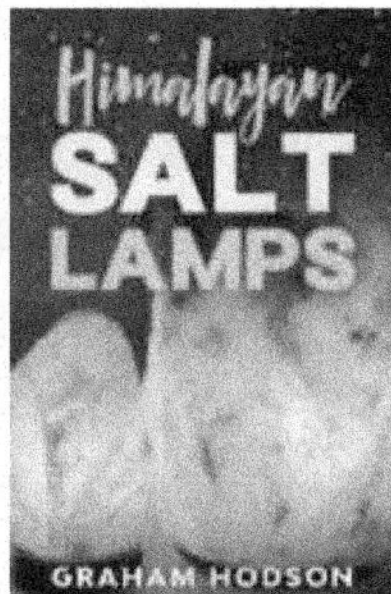

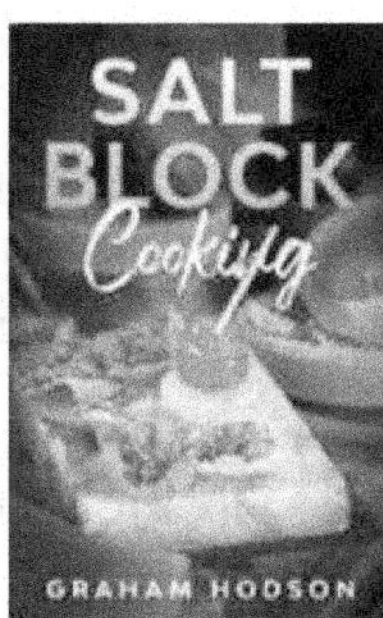

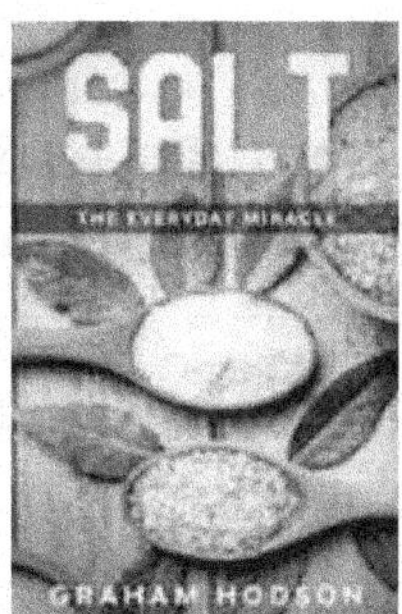

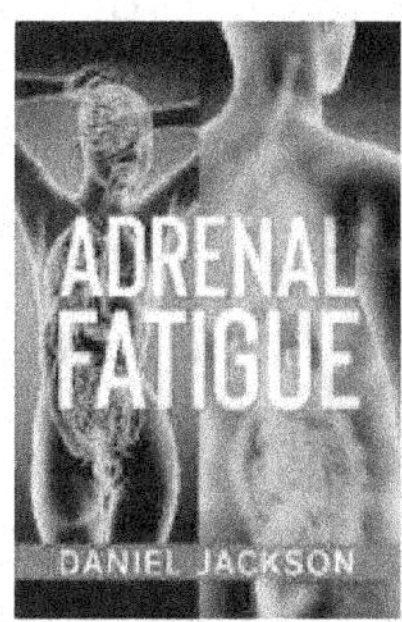

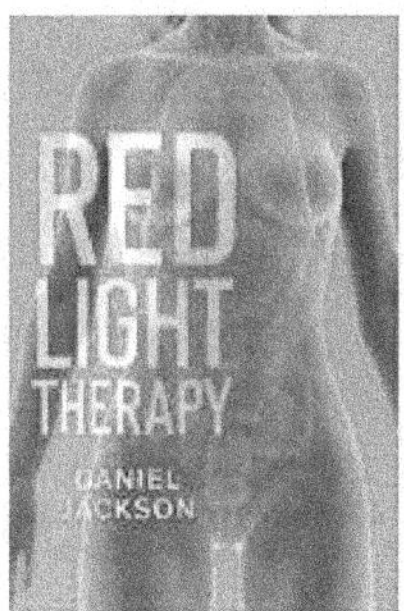

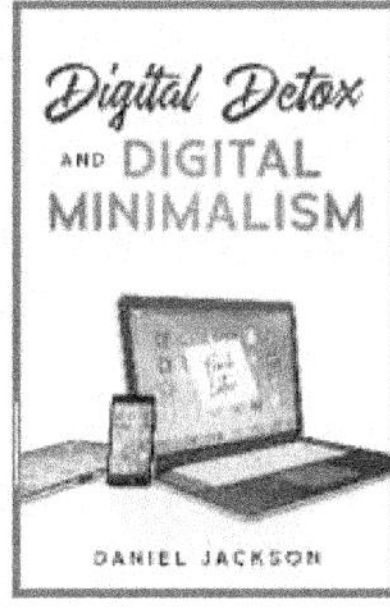

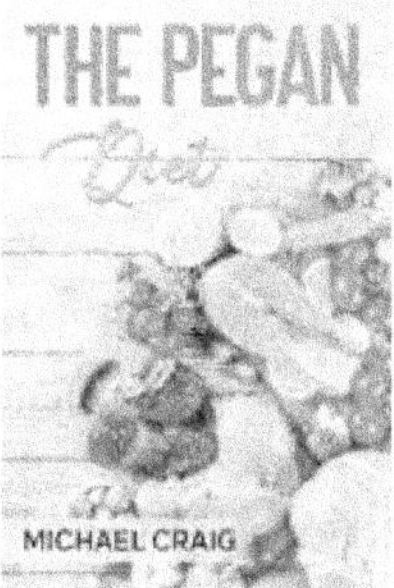

Take a look at more great books available from Rockwood Publishing

… some for **FREE!**

Just visit the link below:

rockwoodpublishing.co.uk

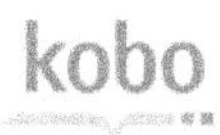
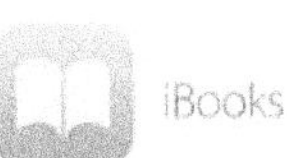
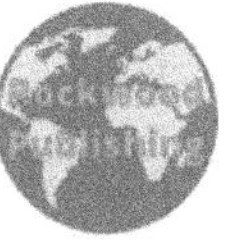
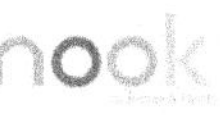
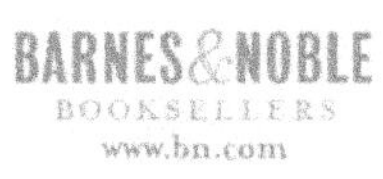

unavailable or being removed from the Internet. The accuracy and completeness of the information provided herein and opinions stated herein are not guaranteed or warranted to produce any particular results, and the advice and strategies contained herein may not be suitable for every individual. The author shall not be liable for any loss incurred as a consequence of the use and application, directly or indirectly, of any information presented in this work. This publication is designed to provide information in regards to the subject matter covered. The information included in this book has been compiled to give an overview of the subject(s) and detail some of the symptoms, treatments etc. that are available to people with this condition. It is not intended to give medical advice. For a firm diagnosis of your condition, and for a treatment plan suitable for you, you should consult your doctor or consultant. The writer of this book and the publisher are not responsible for any damages or negative consequences following any of the treatments or methods highlighted in this book. Website links are for informational purposes and should not be seen as a personal endorsement; the same applies to the products detailed in this book. The reader should also be aware that although the web links included were correct at the time of writing, they may become out of date in the future.

Disclaimers

The content contained within this book is for information and entertainment purposes only, and in no way purports to represent professional medical opinion. It should NOT be used as a substitute for expert advice, and you must consult with your designated health professional before acting upon any information contained herein or before undertaking any practice whose methodology is referred to in this book. The author is NOT a registered health professional and the text merely represents personal opinion, not medical fact. The author cannot be held responsible for the consequences of any action derived from the reading of this book, as the content is not based on diagnosis and subsequent regimen. It is the reader's responsibility to seek proper, professional medical advice from a registered health practitioner in connection with any material contained within this book.

Legal Disclaimer (part 1)

Nothing in this book should be construed as an attempt to diagnose, treat or cure. The information in this book is intended to be a community resource. The author takes no responsibility for any informational material or brochures produced using information taken from this book. The author has endeavoured to ensure that all information is correct at the time of publication. This information, however, is subject to change without notice. The author makes no warranty concerning the accuracy of any information and will not be liable for any errors or omissions. Any liability that arises as a result of this information is hereby excluded to the fullest extent allowed by law.

This information should not be used as a substitute for seeking independent professional advice.

Legal Disclaimer (part 2)

Disclaimer and Terms of Use:

a) i. In publishing this information, the author makes no representations concerning the efficacy, appropriateness or suitability of any products or treatments. Use this information at your own risk. The compiler is not a doctor and has no medical background or training.

ii. Statements and information regarding dietary supplements, books and any products mentioned have not been evaluated by any health authority and are not intended to diagnose, treat, cure or prevent any disease or health condition.

b) In view of the possibility of human error, neither the author nor any other party involved in providing this information, warrant that the information contained therein is in every respect accurate or complete and they are not responsible nor liable for any errors or omissions that may be found or for the results obtained from the use of such information. The entire risk as to the use of this information is assumed by the user.

c) You are encouraged to consult other sources and confirm the information.

d) The information you access is provided "as is". No warranty, expressed or implied, is given as to the accuracy, completeness or timeliness of any information herein, or for obtaining legal advice. To the fullest extent permissible according to applicable law, neither the author nor any other parties who have been involved in the creation, preparation, printing, or delivering of this information assume responsibility for the completeness, accuracy, timeliness, errors or omissions of said information and assume no liability for any direct, incidental, consequential, indirect, or punitive damages as well as any circumstance for any complication, injuries, side effects or other medical accidents to person or property arising from or in connection with the use or reliance upon any information contained herein.

e) The author is not responsible for the contents of any linked site or any link contained in a linked site, or any changes or update to such sites. The inclusion of any link does not imply endorsement by the author. The author makes no representations or claims as to the quality, content and accuracy of the information, services, products, messages which may be provided by such resources, and specifically disclaims any warranties, including but not limited to implied or express warranties of merchantability or fitness for any particular usage, application or purpose.

f) The information provided is general in nature and is intended for educational and informational purposes only. It is not intended to replace or substitute the evaluation, judgment, diagnosis, and medical or preventative care of a physician, paediatrician, therapist and/or health care provider.

g) Any medical, nutritional, dietetic, therapeutic or other decisions, dosages, treatments or drug regimes should be made in consultation with a health care practitioner. Do not discontinue treatment or medication without first consulting your physician, clinician or therapist.

h) By reading this information, you signify your assent to these terms and conditions of use. If you do not agree to these terms and conditions of use, do not read/use this information. If any provision of these terms and conditions of use shall be determined to be unlawful, void or for any reason unenforceable, then that provision shall be deemed severable from this agreement and shall not affect the validity and enforceability of any remaining provisions.

i) The information, services, products, messages and other materials, individually and collectively, are provided with the understanding that the author is not engaged in rendering medical advice or recommendations.

j) The information and the terms of use are subject to change without notice. The material provided as is without warranty of any kind and may include inaccuracies and/or typographical errors. The author makes no representations about the suitability of this information for any purpose. The author disclaims all warranties with regard to this information, including all implied warranties, and in no event shall the author be held liable, resulting from, or in any way related to, the use of this information.

k) The unauthorized alteration of the content of this information is expressly prohibited. The author, its agents and representatives shall not be responsible for any claims, actions or damages which may arise on account of the unauthorized alteration of this information.